Keto diet recipes

for women over 50

Reboot your metabolism with quick and

easy recipes

for losing weight with taste.

By Matilda Fox

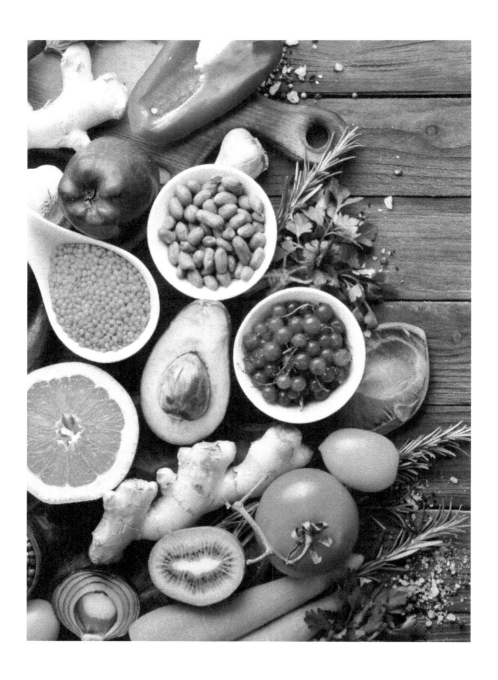

as such, any inattention, use, or misuse of the information in question by the reader will render any resulting actions solely under their purview. There are no scenarios in which the publisher or the original author of this work can be in any fashion deemed liable for any hardship or damages that may befall them after undertaking information described herein.

Additionally, the information in the following pages is intended only for informational purposes and should thus be thought of as universal. As befitting its nature, it is presented without assurance regarding its prolonged validity or interim quality. Trademarks that are mentioned are done without written consent and can in no way be considered an endorsement from the trademark holder.

Table of contents

Introduction

Women go through so much in life, don't we? From growing up, discovering the joys of life, pursuing a promising career, becoming a mother, there is so much that changes within such a short period.

While that is a part of life, what anyone would genuinely try and avoid would be putting on excessive weight that we carry around like unneeded luggage. It is embarrassing, it is distracting, and it is causing quite a few internal issues.

If you thought the biggest hurdle you will face when you hit 50 is a big belly, think again. It isn't the only problem we face. While some would say that having a generous belly is the biggest problem, we firmly believe that there are more serious issues to worry about than that. When it comes to women, well, things aren't looking good.

Our bodies, since birth, continuously change. Most of these changes do not harm us and are only natural. However, once we enter into our 50s, things are a lot different. Now, any changes within our body will directly affect how we perform, operate, and work. If we were to keep these changes unchecked and pay no close attention, things would take a worse turn.

Most of these issues will remain the same for men; however, due to our bodies' chemistry and differences, both internal and external, both would face a variety of issues exclusive to their gender. There are a few ways we can avoid these issues. Some of these ways require you to go back in time, start working out from a very young age, control your diet, and change your habits. That is the stuff of science fiction and hence is out of the equation.

Other ways would include visiting a doctor and getting pills and energy boosters to feel better while taking more pills to fight diabetes, high blood pressure, and other health issues. This way is not just hectic but far too complicated as well.

For a very long time, the only other way was to avoid worrying too much and hope that life would fix issues itself, and that never ended well for many. People have then left with worry and a gap that nothing was able to fill. In comes ketogenic diet. Call it a need of the hour, a savior in disguise, or anything you like. The fact remains that this is proving to be a popular option that is not only delivering results but is also helping millions to maintain a healthy lifestyle and reverse some of the damage their bodies have suffered.

Numerous studies have supported the idea that keto diets are far more effective for older men and women than the younger folks. With so much to look forward to and so little to sacrifice, it does make sense to state that Keto is essentially becoming your permanent way of life once you hit 50. But why is that? Why do we proclaim Keto as an important lifestyle choice for women above 50?

The answer to this involves some explanation; as a woman, you have likely experienced significant differences in how you must diet compared to how men can diet. Women tend to have a harder time losing weight because of their different hormones and how their bodies break down fats. Another factor to consider is your age group. As the body ages, it is important to be more attentive to how you care for yourself. Aging bodies start to experience problems more quickly, which can be avoided with the proper diet and exercise plan. Keto works well for women of all ages, and this is because of how it communicates with the body. No matter how fit your body is right now or how much weight you need or want to lose, Keto will change the way that your body metabolizes, giving you a very personalized experience.

When starting your Keto diet, you should not be thinking about extremes because that isn't what Keto should be about. You should be able to place your body into ketosis without feeling terrible in the process. One of the biggest guidelines to follow while starting your Keto journey is to listen to your body regularly. If you ever think that you are starving or simply unfulfilled, you will likely have to modify the way you are eating because it isn't reaching ketosis properly. It is not an overnight journey, so you need to remember to be patient with yourself and your body. Adapting to a Keto diet takes a bit of transition time and a lot of awareness.

The health benefits of the Keto diet are not different for men or women, but the speed at which they are reached does differ. As mentioned, women's bodies are a lot different when it comes to burning fats and losing weight. For example, by design, women have at least 10% more body fat than men. No matter how fit you are, this is just an aspect of being a woman you must consider. Don't be hard on yourself if you notice that it seems like men can lose weight easier — that's because they can! What women have in additional body fat, men typically have the same in muscle mass. It is why men tend to see faster external results. That added muscle mass means that their metabolism rates are higher. That increased metabolism means that fat and energy get burned more quickly. When you are on Keto, though, the internal change is happening right away.

Your metabolism is unique, but it will also be slower than a man's by nature. Since muscle can burn more calories than fat, the weight seems to fall off men, giving them the ability to reach muscle growth quickly. It should not be something that holds you back from starting your Keto journey. As long as you keep these realistic bodily factors in mind, you won't be left wondering why it takes you a little longer to start losing weight. This point will come for you, but it will take a bit more of a process you must be committed to following through with.

A woman can experience another unique condition, but a man cannot be PCOS or Polycystic Ovary Syndrome, a hormonal imbalance that causes cysts' development. These cysts can cause pain, interfere with normal reproductive function, and burst in extreme and dangerous cases. PCOS is very common among women, affecting up to 10% of the entire female population. Surprisingly, most women are not even aware that they have the condition. Around 70% of women have PCOS, which is undiagnosed. This condition can cause a significant hormonal imbalance, therefore affecting your metabolism. It can also inevitably lead to weight gain, making it even harder to see results while following diet plans. To stay on top of your health, you must make sure that you are going to the gynecologist regularly.

Menopause is another reality that must be faced by women, especially as we age. Most women begin the process of menopause in their mid-40s. Men do not go through menopause, so they are spared from another condition that causes slower metabolism and weight gain. When you start menopause, it is easy to gain weight and lose muscle. Once menopause begins, most women lose muscle faster and conversely gain weight, despite dieting and exercise regimens. Keto can, therefore, be the right diet plan for you. Regardless of what your body is doing naturally, via processes like menopause, your internal systems are still going to be making the switch from running on carbs to deriving energy from fats. When the body begins to run on fats successfully, you have an automatic fuel reserve waiting to be burned. It will take time for your body to do this. However, when it does, you will eat fewer calories and still feel full because your body knows to take energy from the fat you already have. It will become automatic. However, it is a process that requires some patience, but being aware of what is going on with your body can help you stay motivated while on Keto.

Because a Keto diet reduces the amount of sugar you are consuming, it naturally lowers insulin in your bloodstream. It can have amazing effects on any existing PCOS and fertility issues and menopausal symptoms and conditions like pre-diabetes and Type 2 diabetes. Once your body adjusts to a Keto diet, you are overcoming the naturally in place that can prevent you from losing weight and getting healthy. Even if you placed your body on a strict diet, if it isn't getting rid of sugars properly, you likely aren't going to see the same results you will when you try Keto. It is a big reason why Keto can be so beneficial for women.

For women over 50, there are guidelines to follow when you start your Keto diet. As long as you follow the method properly and listen to what your body truly needs, you should have no more problems than men do while following the plan. What you will have are more obstacles to overcome, but you can do it. Remember that plenty of women successfully follow a Keto diet and see great results. Use these women as inspiration for how you anticipate your journey to go. When it seems impossible, remember what you have working against you, but more importantly, what you have working for you. Your body is designed to go into ketogenesis more than designed to store fat by overeating carbs. Use this as inspiration or motivation to keep pushing you ahead. Keto is a valid option for you, and the results will prove this, especially if you are over the age of 50.

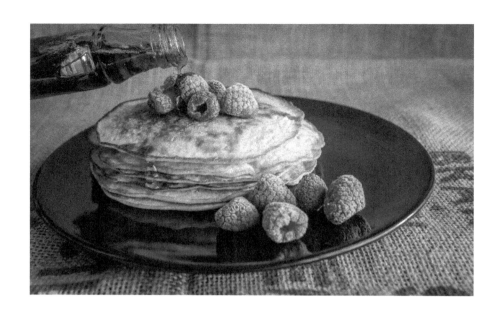

Chapter. 1

Breakfast

1. Taco Egg Muffins

Preparation Time: 10 minutes

Cooking Time: 30 minutes

Servings: 8

Ingredients:

- ½ pound Ground beef, grass-fed
- 1 ½ tablespoon Taco seasoning
- 1 tablespoon salted butter, melted

- 3 Eggs, organic
- 3 ounces Mexican cheese blend, shredded and full-fat
- ½ cup Tomato salsa, organic

Directions:

1. Set oven to 350 degrees F and preheat.
2. Meanwhile, place a skillet pan over medium heat, grease with oil and when hot, add ground beef and cook for 7 minutes or more until almost cooked.
3. Season beef with the taco seasoning and cook for 3 to 5 minutes or until cooked through, then remove the pan from heat.
4. Crack eggs in a bowl, whisk until beaten, then add cooked taco beef along with 2 ounces of Mexican cheese and whisk until well combined.
5. Take a 32 cups muffin pan or parchment-lined silicone muffin cups, grease each cup with melted butter, then evenly fill with taco beef mixture and top with remaining cheese.
6. Bake within 20 minutes or until muffins are cooked through, and the top is nicely golden brown.

7. When done, let muffins cool in the pan for 10 minutes, then take them out and cool on a wire rack. Serve muffins with salsa.

Nutrition:

Calories: 329

Fat: 22.15 g

Protein: 25.2 g

Carbs: 1.8 g

Fiber: 1.2 g;

2. Chocolate Protein Pancakes

Preparation Time: 10 minutes

Cooking Time: 15 minutes

Servings: 12

Ingredients:

- 1/2 cup Almond flour, blanched
- 1/2 cup Whey protein powder
- 1 teaspoon Baking powder
- 1/8 tsp Sea salt
- 3 tablespoons Erythritol sweetener
- 1 teaspoon Vanilla extract, unsweetened
- 3 tablespoons Cocoa powder, organic, unsweetened
- 4 Eggs, pastured
- 2 tablespoons Avocado oil
- 1/3 cup Almond milk, unsweetened

Directions:

1. Put all the fixings in a large mixing bowl, beat using an immersion blender or until well combined, and then let the mixture stand for 5 minutes.
2. Then take a medium skillet pan, place it over medium-low heat, grease it with avocado oil and

pour in prepared pancake batter in small circles of about 3-inches diameter.

3. Cover the skillet pan with lid, let the pancakes cook for 3 minutes or until bubbles form on top, then flip them and continue cooking for 1 to 2 minutes or until nicely golden brown.

4. Cook remaining pancakes in the same manner; you will end up with 12 pancakes, and then let them cool at room temperature.

5. Place cooled pancakes in a freezer bag, with parchment sheet between them, and freeze them for up to 3 months or store in the refrigerator for 5 to 7 days.

6. When ready to serve, and microwave pancakes for 30 seconds to 1 minute or bake in the oven for 5 minutes until thoroughly heated.

Nutrition:

Calories: 237

Fat: 20 g

Protein: 11 g

Carbs: 5 g

Fiber: 2 g;

3. Frittata

Preparation Time: 5 minutes

Cooking Time: 17 minutes

Servings: 1

Ingredients:

- 5 ounces Bacon slices, pastured, diced
- 1/2 medium red onion, peeled, diced
- 1/2 Red bell pepper, cored, diced
- 1/4 teaspoon salt
- 1 teaspoon ground black pepper
- 3 tablespoons Avocado oil
- 1/4 cup and 2 tbsp Grated parmesan cheese, full-fat
- 6 Eggs, pastured

Directions:

1. Take an 8 inches skillet pan, grease with oil, and place it over medium heat.
2. Add onion, pepper, and bacon, cook for 5 minutes or until slightly golden, and then season with salt and black pepper.
3. Beat the eggs in a bowl, add ¼ cup cheese until combined.

4. When bacon is cooked, pour the egg mixture into the pan, spread evenly, and cook for 5 minutes or until frittata is set.
5. In the meantime, switch on the broiler and let preheat. When the frittata is set, sprinkle remaining cheese on the top, then place the pan under the broiler and cook for 4 minutes or until golden brown.
6. Let the frittata cool at room temperature, then cut it into four pieces, place each frittata piece in a heatproof glass meal prep container and store them in the refrigerator for 5 to 7 days.
7. When ready to serve, microwave frittata in their container for 1 to 2 minutes or until thoroughly heated.

Nutrition:

Calories: 494

Fat: 40 g

Protein: 32 g

Carbs: 2.9 g

Fiber: 0.1 g;

4. Bacon and Zucchini Muffins

Preparation Time: 10 minutes

Cooking Time: 35 minutes

Servings: 8

Ingredients:

- 2 cups grated zucchini
- 1 Green onion, chopped
- 2 thyme sprigs leave removed
- 1/2 cup Coconut flour
- 7 Eggs, pastured
- 1/2 teaspoon salt
- 1 teaspoon ground turmeric
- 5 Slices of bacon, pastured, diced
- 1 teaspoon Baking powder
- 1/2 tablespoon Apple cider vinegar
- 1 scoop collagen peptides

Directions:

1. Prepare your oven to 350 F to preheat.
2. Take a medium frying pan, place it over medium heat, add bacon pieces, and cook for 3 to 5 minutes until crispy.
3. Then transfer cooked bacon in a large bowl, add remaining ingredients and stir until well combined.

4. Take an eight cups silicon muffin tray, grease the cups with avocado oil, and then evenly scoop the prepared batter in them.
5. Bake the muffins within 30 minutes or until thoroughly cooked, and the top is nicely golden brown.
6. When done, take out muffins from the tray and cool on the wire rack.
7. Place muffins in a large freezer bag or wrap each muffin with foil and store them in the refrigerator.
8. When ready to serve, microwave muffins for 45 seconds to 1 minute or until thoroughly heated.

Nutrition:

Calories: 104

Fat: 7.2 g

Protein: 7.9 g

Carbs: 1.5 g

Fiber: 0.9 g;

5 Blueberry Pancake Bites

Preparation Time: 10 minutes

Cooking Time: 25 minutes

Servings: 24

Ingredients:

- 1/2 cup frozen blueberries
- 1/2 cup Coconut flour
- 1 teaspoon Baking powder
- 1/2 teaspoon salt
- 1/4 cup Swerve Sweetener
- 1/4 teaspoon Cinnamon
- 1/2 teaspoon Vanilla extract, unsweetened
- 1/4 cup Butter, grass-fed, unsalted, melted
- 4 Eggs, pastured
- 1/3 cup Water

Directions:

1. Set oven to 350 degrees F and let preheat until muffins are ready to bake.
2. Crack the eggs in a bowl, add vanilla and sweetener, whisk using an immersion blender until blended, and then blend in salt, cinnamon, butter, baking powder, and flour until incorporated and smooth batter comes.

3. Let the batter sit within 10 minutes or until thickened and then blend in water until combined.
4. Take a 25 cups silicone mini-muffin tray, grease the cups with avocado oil, then evenly scoop the prepared batter in them and top with few blueberries, pressing the berries gently into the batter.
5. Bake the muffins within 25 minutes or until thoroughly cooked, and the top is nicely golden brown.
6. When done, take out muffins from the tray and cool them on the wire rack.
7. Place muffins in a large freezer bag or evenly divide them into packets and store them in the refrigerator for four days or in the freezer for up to 3 months.
8. When ready to serve, microwave the muffins for 45 seconds to 1 minute or until thoroughly heated.

Nutrition:

Calories: 188

Fat: 13.8 g

Protein: 5.7 g

Carbs: 3.8 g

Fiber: 3.7 g

6. Pretzels

Preparation Time: 10 minutes
Cooking Time: 12 minutes
Servings: 6
Ingredients:
- 1 1/2 cups Almond flour, blanched
- 1/2 teaspoon Coconut sugar
- 1 tablespoon Baking powder
- 1/4 teaspoon Xanthan gum
- 2 1/4 teaspoon dry yeast, active
- 1/4 cup water, lukewarm
- 2 Eggs, Pastured, beaten
- 3 cups Mozzarella cheese, full-fat, shredded
- 2 ounces Cream cheese, full-fat, cubed
- 1 teaspoon salt

Directions:
1. Put yeast in a small bowl, add sugar, pour in water, stir until just mixed and let it sit at a warm place for 10 minutes or until frothy.
2. Then pour the yeast mixture into a food processor, add flour, xanthan gums, eggs, baking powder, and pulse for 1 to 2 minutes or until well combined.
3. Take a heatproof bowl, add cream cheese and mozzarella, and microwave for 2 minutes or until melted, stirring every 30 seconds until smooth.
4. Add melted cheese into the processed flour mixture and continue blending until the dough comes, scraping the mixture from the blender's sides frequently.

5. Transfer the dough into a bowl and then place it in the refrigerator for 20 minutes or until chilled.
6. Meanwhile, set the oven to 400 degrees F and let preheat. Take out the chilled dough from the refrigerator, then divide the dough into six parts and shape each piece into a bowl, using oiled hands.
7. Working on one part at a time, first, roll the piece into an 18-inches long log, then take one end, loop it around and down across the bottom and loop the other end, in the same manner, crossing over the first loop to form a pretzel.
8. Prepare remaining pretzels in the same manner and place them on a baking sheet lined with parchment sheet.
9. Sprinkle salt over pretzels, pressing down lightly, then place the baking sheet into the oven and bake pretzels for 10 to 12 minutes until nicely golden.
10. When done, cool the pretzels at room temperature, then keep them in a large plastic bag and store in the refrigerator for up to a week or freeze for up to 3 months.
11. When ready to serve, bake the pretzels at 400 degrees F for 6 to 7 minutes until hot.

Nutrition:
Calories: 370
Fat: 28 g
Protein: 23 g
Carbs: 6 g
Fiber: 3 g

7. Spiced Butter Waffles

Preparation time: 15 minutes

Cooking time: 20 minutes

Servings: 4

Ingredients:

- ½ cup super fine almond flour
- ½ teaspoon Erythritol
- ¼ teaspoon organic baking powder
- ¼ teaspoon baking soda
- ¼ teaspoon ground cinnamon
- 1/8 teaspoon ground cloves
- 1/8 teaspoon ground nutmeg
- ¼ teaspoon salt
- 2 organic eggs (whites and yolks separated)
- 2 tablespoons butter, melted
- 1 teaspoon organic vanilla extract

Directions:

1. Add flour, Erythritol, baking powder, baking soda, spices, and salt in a mixing bowl and mix well.
2. In a second bowl, add the egg yolks, butter, vanilla, and beat until well combined. In a third small glass bowl, add the egg whites and beat until soft peaks form.

—

3. Add the egg yolks mixture into the flour mixture and mix until well combined. Gently fold in the beaten egg whites.
4. Warm the waffle iron and then grease it. Place ¼ of the mixture into preheated waffle iron and cook for about 4–5 minutes or until golden brown.
5. Repeat with the remaining mixture. Serve warm.

Nutrition:

Calories 177

Fat 15.5 g

Cholesterol 97 mg

Sodium 299 mg

Carbs 3.1 g

Fiber 1.6 g

Sugar 0.8 g

Protein 2.8 g

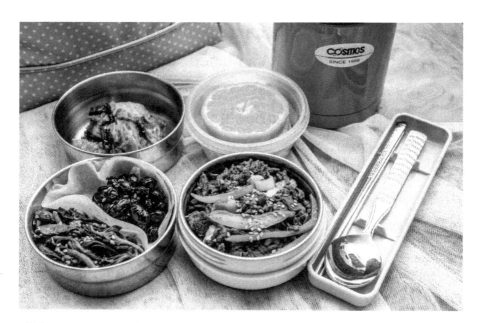

Chapter 2

Lunch

8. Tuna Burgers

Preparation time: 15 minutes

Cooking time: 6 minutes

Servings: 2

Ingredients:

- 1 (15-ounce) can water-packed tuna, drained
- ½ celery stalk, chopped
- 2 tablespoon fresh parsley, chopped
- 1 teaspoon fresh dill, chopped

- 2 tablespoons walnuts, chopped
- 2 tablespoons mayonnaise
- 1 organic egg, beaten
- 1 tablespoon butter
- 3 cups lettuce

Directions:

1. For burgers: Add all ingredients (except the butter and lettuce) in a bowl and mix until well combined. Make 2 equal-sized patties from the mixture.
2. Dissolve the butter over medium heat in a frying pan and cook the patties for about 2–3 minutes.
3. Carefully flip the side and cook for about 2–3 minutes. Divide the lettuce onto serving plates. Top each dish with 1 burger and serve.

Nutrition:

Calories 631

Fat 39.9 g

Cholesterol 168 mg

Sodium 279 mg

Carbs 4.1 g

Fiber 0.3 g

Sugar 1.2 g

Protein 61.7 g

9. Beef Burgers

Preparation time: 15 minutes

Cooking time: 6 minutes

Servings: 2

Ingredients:

- 8 ounces grass-fed ground beef
- Salt and ground black pepper, as required
- 1-ounce mozzarella cheese, cubed
- 1 tablespoon unsalted butter
- Yogurt Sauce:
- 1/3 cup plain Greek yogurt
- 1 teaspoon fresh lemon juice
- ¼ teaspoon garlic, minced
- Salt, as required
- ½ teaspoon granulated erythritol

Directions:

1. In a bowl, add the beef, salt, and black pepper, and mix until well combined. Make 2 equal-sized patties from the mixture.
2. Place mozzarella cube inside of each patty and cover with the beef. In a frying pan, melt butter over medium heat and cook the patties for about 2–3 minutes per side.

3. Divide the greens onto serving plates and top each with 1 patty.
4. Meanwhile, for the yogurt sauce: place all the ingredients in a serving bowl and mix it well. Divide patties onto each serving plate and serve alongside the yogurt sauce.

Nutrition:

Calories 322

Fat 19.8 g

Cholesterol 100 mg

Sodium 308 mg

Carbs 3.5 g

Fiber 0 g

Sugar 2.9 g

Protein 29.5 g

10. Lamb Meatballs

Preparation time: 20 minutes
Cooking time: 1 hour 10 minutes
Servings: 6
Ingredients:
Tomato Chutney:
- 2 cups tomatoes, chopped
- 2 tablespoons fresh red chili, chopped
- 1 tablespoon fresh ginger, peeled and chopped
- ½ tablespoon fresh lime zest, grated
- ¼ cup organic apple cider vinegar
- 2 tablespoons red boat fish sauce
- 1 tablespoon fresh lime juice
- 2 tablespoons granulated erythritol
- ¼ teaspoon mustard powder
- ½ teaspoon dehydrated onion flakes
- ½ teaspoon ground coriander
- ½ teaspoon ground cinnamon
- ¼ teaspoon ground allspice
- 1/8 teaspoon ground cloves
- Salt, as required

Meatballs:
- 1-pound grass-fed ground lamb
- 1 tablespoon olive oil
- 1 teaspoon dehydrated onion flakes, crushed
- ½ teaspoon granulated garlic
- ½ teaspoon ground cumin
- ½ teaspoon red pepper flakes, crushed
- Salt, as required

Directions:
1. For the chutney: Add all the ingredients in a pan over medium heat (except for cilantro) and boil. Adjust the heat to low and simmer for about 45 minutes, stirring occasionally. Remove from heat and set aside to cool.

---

2. Meanwhile, preheat your oven to 400ºF. Line a larger baking sheet with parchment paper.
3. For meatballs: In a large bowl, place all the ingredients, and with your hands, mix until well combined. Shape the mixture into desired and equal-sized balls.
4. Arrange meatballs into the prepared baking sheet in a single layer and bake for about 15–20 minutes or until done completely. Serve the meatballs with chutney.

Nutrition:
Calories 184
Fat 8.1 g
Cholesterol 68 mg
Sodium 586 mg
Carbs 3.5 g
Fiber 1 g
Sugar 1.9 g
Protein 23.3 g

11. Stuffed Zucchini

Preparation time: 15 minutes

Cooking time: 18 minutes

Servings: 8

Ingredients:

- 4 medium zucchinis, halved lengthwise
- 1 cup red bell pepper, seeded and minced
- ½ cup Kalamata olives, pitted and minced
- ½ cup fresh tomatoes, minced
- 1 teaspoon garlic, minced
- 1 tablespoon dried oregano, crushed
- Salt and ground black pepper, as required
- ½ cup feta cheese, crumbled

Directions:

1. Preheat your oven to 350ºF. Grease a large baking sheet.
2. Scoop each zucchini half, then discard the flesh.
3. In a bowl, mix the bell pepper, olives, tomatoes, garlic, oregano, salt, and black pepper.
4. Stuff each zucchini half with the veggie mixture evenly. Arrange zucchini halves onto the prepared baking sheet and bake for about 15 minutes.

5. Now, set the oven to broiler on high. Top each zucchini half with feta cheese and broil for about 3 minutes. Serve hot.

Nutrition:

Calories 59

Fat 3.2 g

Cholesterol 8 mg

Sodium 208 mg

Carbs 6.2 g

Fiber 0.9 g

Sugar 3.2 g

Protein 2.9 g

12. Stuffed Bell Peppers

Preparation time: 15 minutes

Cooking time: 20 minutes

Servings: 6

Ingredients:

- 2 teaspoons coconut oil
- 1-pound grass-fed ground beef
- 1 garlic clove, minced
- 1 cup white mushrooms, chopped
- 1 cup yellow onion, chopped
- Salt and ground black pepper, as required
- ½ cup homemade tomato puree
- 3 large green bell peppers, halved
- 1 cup of water
- 4 ounces sharp cheddar cheese, shredded

Directions:

1. Dissolve the coconut oil in a wok over medium-high heat and sauté the garlic for about 30 seconds.
2. Add the beef and cook for about 5 minutes, crumbling with the spoon. Add the mushrooms and onion and cook for about 5–6 minutes.

3. Stir in salt and black pepper and cook for about 30 seconds. Remove, then stir in the tomato puree.
4. Meanwhile, in a microwave-safe dish, arrange the bell peppers, cut-side down. Pour the water into the baking dish.
5. With a plastic wrap, cover the baking dish and microwave on high for about 4–5 minutes. Remove from microwave and uncover the baking dish.
6. Drain the water completely. Now in the baking dish, arrange the bell peppers, cut-side up.
7. Stuff the bell peppers evenly with beef mixture and top with cheese. Microwave on High for about 2–3 minutes. Serve warm.

Nutrition:

Calories 258

Fat 15.4 g

Cholesterol 70 mg

Sodium 206 mg

Carbs 8 g

Fiber 2.3 g

Sugar 4.1 g

Protein 21.8 g

13. Spinach in Creamy Sauce

Preparation time: 10 minutes

Cooking time: 15 minutes

Servings: 4

Ingredients:

- 2 tablespoons unsalted butter
- 1 small yellow onion, chopped
- 1 cup cream cheese, softened
- 2 packages frozen spinach, thawed
- 2–3 tablespoons water
- Salt and ground black pepper, as required
- 1 teaspoon fresh lemon juice

Directions:

1. Dissolve the butter in a wok over medium heat and sauté the onion for about 6–8 minutes.
2. Add the cream cheese and cook for about 2 minutes or until melted completely.
3. Stir in the spinach and water and cook for about 4–5 minutes. Stir in the salt, black pepper, and lemon juice, and remove from heat. Serve immediately.

Nutrition:

Calories 293

Fat 26.6 g

Cholesterol 79 mg

Sodium 364 mg

Carbs 8.4 g

Fiber 3.5 g

Sugar 1.5 g

Protein 8.7 g

14. Creamy Zucchini Noodles

Preparation time: 15 minutes

Cooking time: 10 minutes

Servings: 6

Ingredients:

- 1¼ cups heavy whipping cream
- ¼ cup mayonnaise
- Salt and ground black pepper, as required
- 30 ounces zucchini, spiralized with blade C
- 3 ounces Parmesan cheese, grated
- 2 tablespoons fresh mint leaves
- 2 tablespoons butter, melted

Directions:

1. In a pan, add the heavy cream and bring to a boil. Lower the heat to low and cook until reduced in half.
2. Add the mayonnaise, salt, and black pepper and cook until the mixture is warm enough. Add the zucchini noodles and gently stir to combine.
3. Stir in the Parmesan cheese and immediately remove from the heat. Divide the zucchini noodles onto 4 serving plates and immediately drizzle with the melted butter. Serve immediately.

Nutrition:

Calories 249

Fat 23.1 g

Cholesterol 58 mg

Sodium 270 mg

Carbs 6.1 g

Fiber 1.7 g

Sugar 2.5 g

Protein 6.9 g

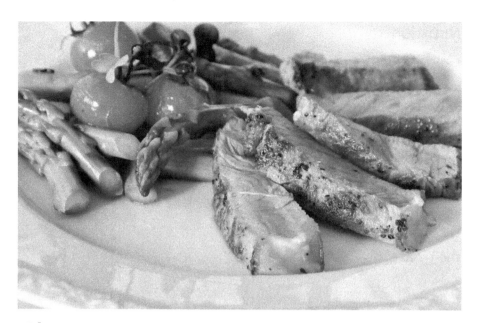

Chapter 3

Dinner

15. Slow Roasting Pork Shoulder

Preparation Time: 15 minutes

Cooking Time: 7 hours

Servings: 8

Ingredients:

- 3 lb. pork shoulder
- 8 garlic cloves, minced
- ½ C. fresh lemon juice

- 2 tbsp. olive oil
- 1 tbsp. low-sodium soy sauce
- 1/3 C. homemade chicken broth

Directions:

1. In a nonreactive baking dish, arrange the pork shoulder, fat side up. With the tip of the knife, score the fat in a crosshatch pattern.
2. In a bowl, add the garlic, lemon juice, soy sauce, and oil and mix well. Place the marinade over pork and coat well.
3. Refrigerate for about 4-6 hours, flipping occasionally. Preheat the oven to 3150 F. Lightly grease a large roasting pan.
4. With paper towels, wipe marinade off the pork shoulder. Arrange the pork shoulder into a prepared roasting pan, fat side up.
5. Roast for about 3 hours. Remove from the oven and pour the broth over the pork shoulder.
6. Roast for about 3-4 hours, basting with pan juices, after every 1 hour. Remove from the oven and place the pork shoulder onto a cutting board for about 30 minutes. Slice and serve.

Nutrition:

Calories: 537

Carbs: 1.5g

Protein: 40.2g

Fat: 40.1g

Sugar: 0.5g

Sodium: 261mg

Fiber: 0.1g

16. Garlicky Pork Shoulder

Preparation Time: 15 minutes

Cooking Time: 6 hours

Servings: 10

Ingredients:

- 1 head garlic, peeled and crushed
- ¼ C. fresh rosemary, minced
- 2 tbsp. fresh lemon juice
- 2 tbsp. balsamic vinegar
- 1 (4-lb.) pork shoulder

Directions:

1. Put all the fixings except pork shoulder in a bowl and mix well. Put the pork shoulder in your roasting pan and generously coat with the marinade.
2. With a large plastic wrap, cover the roasting pan and refrigerate to marinate for at least 1-2 hours.
3. Remove the roasting pan from the refrigerator. Remove the plastic wrap from the roasting pan and keep at room temperature for 1 hour.
4. Preheat the oven to 2750 F. Place the roasting pan into the oven and roast for about 6 hours.
5. Remove from the oven and place pork shoulder onto a cutting board for about 30 minutes. Slice and serve.

Nutrition:

Calories: 502

Carbs: 2g

Protein: 42.5g

Fat: 39.1g

Sugar: 0.1g

Sodium: 125mg

Fiber: 0.7g

17. Rosemary Pork Roast

Preparation Time: 15 minutes

Cooking Time: 1 hour

Servings: 6

Ingredients:

- 1 tbsp. dried rosemary, crushed
- 3 cloves garlic, minced
- Salt
- ground black pepper
- 2 lb. boneless pork loin roast
- ¼ C. olive oil
- 1/3 C. homemade chicken broth

Directions:

1. Preheat the oven to 3500 F, then grease a roasting pan.
2. Put rosemary, garlic, salt, and black pepper in a small bowl and crush it to form a paste.
3. Prick the pork loin at all places, then press the half of rosemary batter into the cuts.
4. Put oil in the bowl with the rest of the rosemary mixture to mix and massage the pork with it.
5. Roast within 1 hour, flipping and coating with the pan juices occasionally.
6. Remove, then transfer the pork to a serving platter. Place the roasting pan over medium heat.

7. Add the broth and cook for about 3-5 minutes, stirring to lose the brown bits. Pour sauce over pork and serve.

Nutrition:

Calories: 294

Carbs: 0.9g

Protein: 40g

Fat: 13.9g

Sugar: 0.1g

Sodium: 156mg

Fiber: 0.3g

18. Winter Season Pork Dish

Preparation Time: 15 minutes

Cooking Time: 2 hours

Servings: 8

Ingredients:

- 24 oz. sauerkraut
- 2 lb. pork roast
- Salt
- ground black pepper
- ¼ C. unsalted butter
- ½ yellow onion, sliced thinly
- 14 oz. precooked kielbasa, cut into ½-inch rounds

Directions:

1. Preheat the oven to 3250 F.
2. Drain the sauerkraut, reserving about 1 C. of liquid. Rub the pork roast with salt plus black pepper.
3. In a heavy-bottomed skillet, melt the butter over high heat and sear the pork for about 5-6 minutes per side.
4. With a slotted spoon, transfer the pork onto a plate. At the bottom of a casserole, place half of sauerkraut and onion slices.
5. Place the seared pork roast and kielbasa pieces on top. Top with the remaining sauerkraut and onion slices.

6. Pour the reserved sauerkraut liquid into the casserole dish. Cover the casserole dish tightly and bake for about 2 hours.
7. Remove from the oven, and with tongs, transfer the pork roast onto a cutting board for at least 15 minutes. With a sharp knife, cut the pork roast into desired size slices.
8. Divide the pork slices onto serving plates and serve alongside the sauerkraut mixture.

Nutrition:

Calories: 417

Carbs: 6.3g

Protein: 39g

Fat: 25g

Sugar: 2g

Sodium: 1200mg

Fiber: 3g

19. Celebrating Pork Tenderloin

Preparation Time: 15 minutes

Cooking Time: 40 minutes

Serves: 6

Ingredients:

For Pork Tenderloin:

- 3 medium garlic cloves, minced
- 3 tsp. dried rosemary, crushed
- ½ tsp. cayenne pepper
- Salt
- ground black pepper
- 2 lb. pork tenderloin

For Blueberry Sauce:

- 1 tbsp. olive oil
- 1 medium yellow onion, chopped
- ½ tsp. Erythritol
- 1/3 C. organic apple cider vinegar
- 1½ C. fresh blueberries
- ½ tsp. dried thyme, crushed
- Salt
- ground black pepper, to taste

Directions:

1. Preheat the oven to 4000 F. Grease a roasting pan.
2. For the pork: in a bowl, mix all the ingredients except pork. Rub the pork with garlic mixture evenly.
3. Place the pork into the prepared roasting pan. Roast for about 25 minutes or until desired doneness.
4. Meanwhile, in a pan, for sauce, heat the oil over medium-high heat and sauté the onion for about 4-5 minutes. Stir in the remaining ingredients and cook for about 7-8 minutes or until desired thickness, stirring frequently.
5. Remove and place the pork tenderloin onto a cutting board for about 10-15 minutes. With a sharp knife, cut the pork tenderloin into desired size slices and serve with the topping of blueberry sauce.

Nutrition:

Calories: 276

Carbs: 9g

Protein: 40g

Fat: 8g

Sugar: 5g

Sodium: 116mg

Fiber: 2g

20. Mustard Pork Tenderloin

Preparation Time: 15 minutes

Cooking Time: 30 minutes

Servings: 4

Ingredients:

- 1 tsp. fresh rosemary, minced
- 1 garlic clove, minced
- 1 tbsp. fresh lemon juice
- 1 tbsp. olive oil
- 1 tsp. Dijon mustard
- 1 tsp. powdered Swerve
- Salt
- ground black pepper
- 1 lb. pork tenderloin
- ¼ C. blue cheese, crumbled

Directions:

1. Preheat oven to 4000 F. Grease a large rimmed baking sheet.
2. Put all the fixings except the pork tenderloin and cheese in a large bowl and beat until well combined.

3. Put the pork tenderloin, then coat with the mixture generously. Arrange the pork tenderloin onto the prepared baking sheet.
4. Bake for about 20-22 minutes. Remove from the oven and place the pork tenderloin onto a cutting board for about 5 minutes.
5. With a sharp knife, cut the pork tenderloin into ¾-inch thick slices and serve with cheese topping.

Nutrition:

Calories: 227

Carbs: 2g

Protein: 37g

Fat: 10g

Sugar: 0.5g

Sodium: 236mg

Fiber: 0.1g

21. Succulent Pork Tenderloin

Preparation Time: 20 minutes

Cooking Time: 1 hour

Servings: 4

Ingredients:

- 1 lb. pork tenderloin
- 1 tbsp. unsalted butter
- 2 tsp. garlic, minced
- 2 oz. fresh spinach
- 4 oz. cream cheese softened
- 1 tsp. liquid smoke
- Salt
- ground black pepper

Directions:

1. Preheat the oven to 3500 F. Line the casserole dish with a piece of the foil.
2. Arrange the pork tenderloin between 2 plastic wraps and with a meat tenderizer, pound until flat. Carefully cut the edges of the tenderloin to shape into a rectangle.
3. Dissolve the butter over medium heat in a large skillet and sauté the garlic for about 1 minute.
4. Add the spinach, cream cheese, liquid smoke, salt, and black pepper and cook for about 3-4 minutes.

5. Remove and set aside to cool slightly. Place the spinach mixture onto pork tenderloin about ½-inch from the edges.
6. Carefully roll tenderloin into a log and secure with toothpicks. Arrange the tenderloin into the prepared casserole dish, seam-side down.
7. Bake for about 1¼ hours. Remove from the oven and let it cool slightly before cutting. Cut the tenderloin into desired sized slices and serve.

Nutrition:

Calories: 315

Carbs: 3g

Protein: 43g

Fat: 23g

Sugar: 0.5g

Sodium: 261mg

Fiber: 0.1g

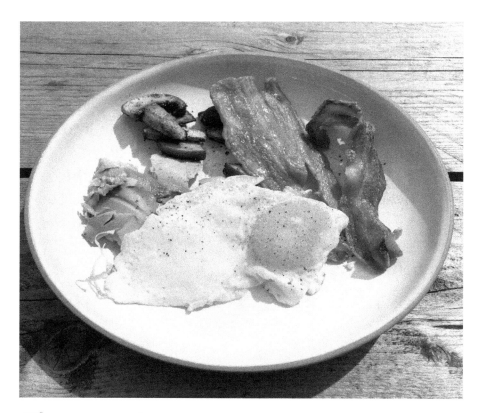

Chapter 4

Snacks

22. Bacon-Wrapped Scallops

Preparation Time: 15 minutes

Cooking Time: 15 minutes

Servings: 4

Ingredients:

- ½ tsp Salt
- ½ tsp Black pepper
- 2 tbsp Olive oil
- 8 slices bacon, cut into half, middle of the slice
- 16 Sea scallops
- 16 Toothpicks

Directions:

1. Heat the oven to 425F. Lay parchment paper on a cookie sheet. Remove any side muscles the scallops might have and dry them with a paper towel.
2. Use one-half of a bacon slice to wrap each scallop around and then hold the bacon to the scallop with a toothpick.
3. Brush on the olive oil and then season it with salt and pepper. Lay the scallops on the parchment paper and bake for fifteen minutes.

Nutrition:

Calories: 224

Carbs: 2g

Fat:17g

Protein: 12g

23. Buffalo Chicken Jalapeno Poppers

Preparation Time: 20 minutes

Cooking Time: 30 minutes

Servings: 5

Ingredients:

- 4 slices cooked bacon
- ¼ cup Buffalo wing sauce
- ¼ cup Shredded Mozzarella cheese
- ½ cup Crumbled Blue cheese
- 4 oz Cream cheese at room temperature
- ½ tsp Salt
- ½ tsp Onion powder
- 2 tbsp minced garlic
- 8 oz Grounded chicken
- 10 large sizes of Jalapeno peppers; cut in half longways and remove the seeds
- Ranch dressing and sliced green onions for serving

Directions:

1. Heat the oven to 350. Lay foil or parchment paper on a cookie sheet. Lay the jalapeno pepper halves on the foil or parchment paper.

2. Cook over medium heat the garlic, ground chicken, onion powder, and salt for about ten minutes until you fully cook the chicken.
3. Put this batter into a big bowl and mix in the wing sauce, mozzarella cheese, and one-quarter cup of the crumbled blue cheese.
4. Put this mix into all the pepper halves and top them with the bacon crumbles and the rest of the blue cheese.
5. Bake the poppers for thirty minutes and serve with the ranch dressing and the green onions.

Nutrition:

Calories: 252

Carbs: 4.6g

Fat: 19g

Protein: 16g

24. Rutabaga Fries

Preparation Time: 15 minutes

Cooking Time: 45 minutes

Servings: 8

Ingredients:

- 24 oz Rutabagas; two medium-sized
- ½ tsp Black pepper
- 1 tsp Salt
- ¼ cup Olive oil

Directions:

1. Heat the oven to 400. Wash and peel the rutabagas and slice them into one-quarter-inch thick circles. Slice each circle into sticks that are one-quarter inch wide.
2. Mix in a big bowl the sticks of rutabaga with the black pepper, salt, and olive oil.
3. Arrange the fries on a metal rack sitting on top of a cookie sheet and back them for forty-five minutes.

Nutrition:

Calories: 96

Carbs: 6g

Fat: 6g

Protein: 1g

25. Spicy Deviled Eggs

Preparation Time: 20 minutes
Cooking Time: 15 minutes
Servings: 24
Ingredients:
- 1 tsp Minced Chives
- 1 tsp Chili powder
- 1 tsp Salt
- 1 tsp Black pepper
- 1 tbsp Dijon mustard
- 1 tbsp Sriracha sauce
- 1/3 cup Mayonnaise
- 12 large Eggs

Directions:

1. Hard boil the eggs, and when they are cool, peel them and cut them in half the long way. Remove the yolks gently and place them into a large bowl.
2. Mash the yolks into a paste with a fork or a potato masher. Stir in the mustard, sriracha sauce, salt, pepper, chili powder, and mayonnaise until the mix is creamy.
3. Refill the white egg with this mixture using a spoon or a frosting bag to pipe the mix. When you are ready to serve the eggs, top them with the chives.

Nutrition:
Calories: 53
Carbs: 1g
Fat: 4g
Protein: 2g

26. Pesto Bacon and Caprese Salad Skewers

Preparation Time: 15 minutes

Cooking Time: 5 minutes

Servings: 10

Ingredients:

- 1 tsp Black pepper
- Salt
- 2 tbsp Olive oil
- ¼ cup Basil pesto
- 30 Mozzarella balls or chunks
- 30 Fresh Basil
- 5 cooked slices bacon, cut into six pieces each
- 30 grape tomatoes
- Toothpicks

Directions:

1. Place the food on the toothpicks in this order: mozzarella balls, basil leaf, bacon piece, and grape tomato.
2. Mix, in a small bowl, the olive oil, the pesto and drizzle it over the skewers, then sprinkle them with salt and pepper.

Nutrition:

Calories: 153

Carbs: 2g

Fat: 12g

Protein: 7g

27. Baked Coconut Shrimp

Preparation Time: 15 minutes

Cooking Time: 10 minutes

Servings: 4

Ingredients:

- ½ tsp Black pepper
- ½ tsp Salt
- ¼ tsp Paprika
- ¼ tsp Garlic powder
- 2 cups of unsweetened coconut flakes
- 3 large Eggs (well beat)
- 3 tbsp Coconut flour
- 1 pound of Thawed Medium shrimp; 42 to 48 peeled and deveined

Directions:

1. Warm the oven to 400 F. Lay a wire rack onto a cookie sheet and spray it with oil spray. Set three bowls on the counter.
2. In the first one, put the beaten eggs; in the other one, put the coconut flakes, and in the last one, put a mix of the pepper, salt, paprika, garlic powder, and coconut flour.
3. Dip each shrimp into the flour mixture first, then into the egg wash, and roll in coconut flakes. Lay them on the wire rack and bake for ten minutes, turning them over after five minutes.

Nutrition:

Calories: 443

Carbs: 5g

Fat: 30g

Protein: 31g

28. Baked Garlic Parmesan Wings

Preparation Time: 15 minutes

Cooking Time: 10 minutes

Servings: 6

Ingredients:

- ½ tsp Black pepper
- 1 tsp Salt
- 1 tsp Onion powder
- 2 tsp Garlic powder
- 1 tbsp Chopped parsley
- 1 tbsp Minced Garlic
- ½ Grated Parmesan cheese
- ½ cup Melted Butter
- 2 tbsp Baking powder
- 2 pounds Thawed chicken wings

Directions:

1. Heat the oven to 250. Salt and pepper the wings and let them sit for ten minutes. Shake the baking powder over the wings and toss them so that the baking powder covers all the wings.
2. Spread the wings on an oven rack and bake them for thirty minutes. Change the temperature of the oven to 425 and bake the wings for another thirty minutes.
3. Prepare the sauce for the wings while the wings are baking by mixing the onion powder, garlic

powder, parsley, minced garlic, parmesan cheese, and melted butter in a bowl.

4. When the wings have finished cooking, let them sit for five minutes and then toss them in the sauce.

Nutrition:

Calories 468

Carbs 2 g

Fat 38 g

Protein 30 g

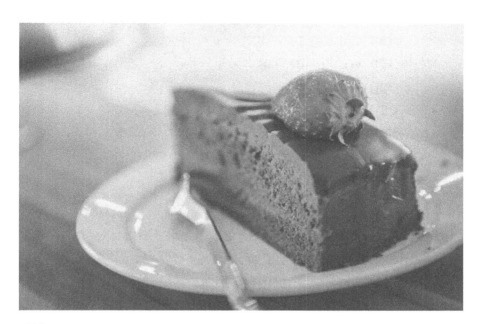

Chapter 5

Dessert

29. Chocolate Mug Muffin

Preparation time: 2 minutes

Cooking time: 2 minutes

Servings: 2

Ingredients:

- 2 tbsp almond four
- 1 tbsp cocoa powder
- 1 tbsp Swerve

- ½ tsp baking powder
- ¼ tsp vanilla extract
- 1 egg
- 1 pinch sea salt
- 1 ½ tbsp melted coconut oil or butter
- ½ ounce sugar-free dark chocolate
- ½ tsp coconut oil

Directions:

1. Mix dry fixings in a small bowl. Stir in egg and melted coconut oil or butter. Mix until smooth.
2. Add coarsely chopped chocolate and pour it into two well-greased coffee mugs—microwave for 90 seconds. Remove and let cool. Serve with a dollop of whipped coconut cream.

Nutrition:

Calories 230

Protein 6g

Fat 21g

Carbs 2g

30. Low Carb Chocolate Mousse

Preparation time: 2 hours

Cooking time: 5 minutes

Servings: 6

Ingredients:

- 1 ¼ cups heavy whipping cream
- ½ tsp vanilla extract
- 2 egg yolks
- 1 pinch sea salt
- 3 ounces dark chocolate with a minimum of 80% cocoa solids

Directions:

1. Chop the chocolate into small pieces, then dissolve in the microwave within 20-second intervals, stirring in between. Set aside at room temperature to cool.
2. Whip the cream to soft peaks, then put the vanilla towards the end. Mix egg yolks plus salt in a different bowl. Add the melted chocolate to the egg yolks and mix to a smooth batter.

3. Add a couple of spoonsful of whipped cream to the chocolate mix and stir to loosen it a bit. Add the remaining cream and fold it through.
4. Divide the batter into ramekins or serving glasses of your choice. Let it chill in the fridge within 2 hours. Serve with fresh berries.

Nutrition:

Calories 270

Protein 3g

Fat 25g

Carbs 6g

31. Strawberry Cheesecake Fat Bombs

Preparation time: 2 hours & 30 minutes

Cooking time: 0 minutes

Servings: 14

Ingredients:

- ½ cup strawberries
- ¾ cup cream cheese softened
- ¼ cup butter
- 2 tbsp powdered erythritol
- ½ teaspoon vanilla extract

Directions:

1. Put the cream cheese plus butter (cut into small pieces) into a mixing bowl. Leave at room temperature for 30 -60 minutes.
2. In the meantime, wash the strawberries and remove the green parts. Place the in a bowl and mash, using a fork or place in a blender for a smooth texture.
3. Mix the powdered erythritol and vanilla extract. Mix the strawberries with the rest of the fixing, make sure they have reached room temperature.
4. Add to the bowl with the softened butter plus cream cheese. Use a food processor and mix well.
5. Put the mixture into small muffin silicon molds. Put in the freezer within 2 hours or until set. Serve.

Nutrition:

Calories 67

Protein 0.96g

Fat 7.4g

Carbs 0.85g

32. Chocolate Chip Cookie Dough Fat Bombs

Preparation time: 60 minutes

Cooking time: 0 minutes

Servings: 12

Ingredients:

- 8 ounces cream cheese, softened
- 1 stick (1/2 cup) salted butter
- ½ cup creamy peanut butter or almond butter
- 1/3 cup swerve sweetener
- 1 tsp vanilla extract
- 4 ounces Stevia sweetened chocolate chips

Directions:

1. Cream everything in a mixer and then spray a cookie scoop with coconut oil cooking spray.
2. Refrigerate dough for 30 minutes before scooping onto parchment paper, then freeze for 30 minutes. Store in refrigerator.

Nutrition:

Calories 139

Protein 2g

Fat 14g

Carbs 2g

33. Keto Tiramisu

Preparation time: 10 minutes

Cooking time: 2 minutes

Servings: 4

Ingredients:

For Filling:

- ½ block of cream cheese (at room temperature)
- ¾ cup heavy whipping cream
- 2 -3 tbsp erythritol

For Mug Cake:

- 3 tbsp almond flour
- 2 tbsp erythritol
- 1 egg
- ½ tsp baking powder
- 1 tsp vanilla extract

Coffee Liquor Mix:

1. 1 shot expresso
2. 1 shot rum
3. Cocoa powder to garnish

Directions:

1. Start by making your coffee mixture. Mix your espresso and rum and place in the fridge for the mixture to get cold.
2. Make Mug cake. Mix all the fixing in a mug and microwave on high within 60 seconds. Remove cake from the mug and let it cool for 5 minutes.

3. Slice the cake into four equal pieces and place them on a cooling rack to cool down completely.
4. For the cream: Mix cream cheese, vanilla extract, and erythritol in a bowl. Mix all fixing until sweetener has completely dissolved, and texture is very smooth using an electric hand mixer.
5. Put heavy whipping cream in a separate bowl and whisk on high speed until medium to stiff peaks forms, about 1 minute. Do not overbeat.
6. Add whipped cream into the cream cheese mixture and mix on low speed within 45 seconds to 1 minute.
7. Dip your sliced almond cake into your coffee mixture. Now place one cake slice on the bottom of the cup/mug you will be serving in, and scoop in 2 tablespoons of the cream filling.
8. Repeat until you build up your tiramisu cup.
9. Put some unsweetened cocoa powder on top, then serve.

Nutrition:

Calories 314

Protein 5g

Fat 29g

Carbs 11.9g

Fiber7.2g

34. No-Bake Keto Mocha Cheesecake

Preparation time: 15 minutes

Cooking time: 0 minutes

Servings: 4

Ingredients:

- ¾ cup heavy whipping cream
- 1 block of cream cheese (room temperature)
- ¼ cup unsweetened cocoa
- ¾ cup Swerve Confectioners sweetener
- 1 double shot of espresso

Directions:

1. Whip the softened cream cheese in a bowl using a hand mixer for 1 minute. Add espresso and continue mixing.
2. Add the sweetener, ¼ cup at a time, and mix. Add cocoa powder and mix until completely blended.
3. Whip the cream in a different bowl until stiff peaks form. Gently fold the whipped cream into the mocha mixture using a spatula—place in individual serving dishes. Enjoy!

Nutrition:

Calories 425

Protein 6g

Fat 33g

Carbs 3.6g

35. Keto Cream Cheese Cookies

Preparation time: 15 minutes

Cooking time: 15 minutes

Servings: 24

Ingredients:

- ¼ cup butter (softened)
- 2 ounces plain cream cheese (softened)
- ½ cup erythritol
- 2 tsp vanilla extract
- 3 cups almond flour
- ¼ tsp sea salt
- 1 large egg white

Directions:

1. Preheat oven to 350°F. Prepare or line a large cookie sheet with parchment paper.
2. Use a hand mixer to beat the butter, cream cheese, and erythritol: beat until fluffy and light in color.
3. Beat in the vanilla extract, salt, and egg white. Beat in almond flour, ½ cup at a time.
4. Use a medium cookie scoop to scoop balls of dough onto the prepared cookie sheet. Flatten with your palm.

5. Bake within 15 minutes, until the edges are lightly golden. Allow cooling completely in the pan before handling (cookies will harden as they cool).

Nutrition:

Calories 106

Protein 3g

Fat 9g

Carbs 3g

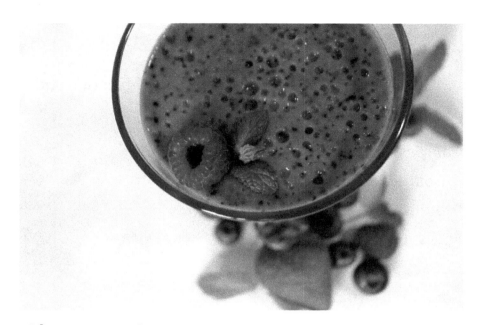

Chapter 6

Smoothies

36. Red Festive Smoothie

Preparation Time: 10 minutes

Cooking time: 0 minutes

Servings: 2

Ingredients:

- ¾ C. raw red beets, chopped
- 4 frozen strawberries
- 2-3 drops liquid stevia
- 1½ C. unsweetened almond milk

- ½ C. ice cubes

Directions:

1. Pulse all the fixing in a high-speed blender until smooth. Serve.

Nutrition:

Calories: 66

Carbs: 9g

Protein: 2g

Fat: 2.8g

Sugar: 5g

Sodium: 184mg

Fiber: 2.8g

37. Pretty Pink Smoothie

Preparation Time: 10 minutes

Cooking time: 0 minutes

Servings: 2

Ingredients:

- ½ c. fresh strawberries, hulled
- 8-10 fresh basil leaves
- 3-4 drops liquid stevia
- ½ C. plain Greek yogurt
- 1 C. unsweetened almond milk
- ¼ C. ice cubes

Directions:

1. In a high-speed blender, add all the fixing and pulse until smooth.
2. Transfer into 2 serving glasses and serve immediately.

Nutrition:

Calories: 75

Carbs: 8g

Protein: 4.3g

Fat: 2.6g

Sugar: 6g

Sodium: 133mg

Fiber: 1.2g

38. Golden Chai Latte Smoothie

Preparation Time: 10 minutes

Cooking time: 0 minutes

Servings: 2

Ingredients:

- 2 tbsp. chia seeds
- 1 tbsp. ground turmeric
- 1 tsp. ground cinnamon
- 1 tsp ground ginger
- ¼ tsp. ground cardamom
- Pinch of ground black pepper
- 2 tbsp. MCT oil
- 2 tsp. stevia powder
- 1¾ C. unsweetened almond milk
- ¼ C. ice cubes

Directions:

1. In a high-speed blender, pulse all the ingredients and pulse until smooth. Serve.

Nutrition:

Calories: 178

Carbohydrates: 8.5g

Protein: 2.7g

Fat: 19.6g

Sugar: 0.2g

Sodium: 137mg

Fiber: 4.8g

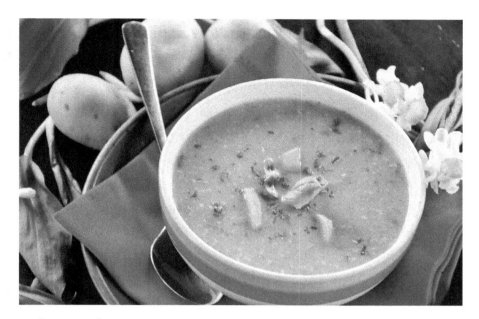

Chapther 7

Soups

39. Spicy Red Curry Roasted Cauliflower Soup

Preparation time: 15 minutes

Cooking time: 40 minutes

Servings: 2

Ingredients:

- 1 tablespoon Thai red curry paste
- ½ large cauliflower, cut into florets

- 2 cups vegetable broth, low sodium
- 1/8 teaspoon Himalayan pink salt
- 7 oz. can coconut milk, unsweetened

Directions:

1. Preheat the oven to 4000F and grease a baking tray.
2. Arrange the cauliflower florets on the baking tray and bake for about 20 minutes.
3. Put the roasted cauliflower and vegetable broth in a blender and blend until smooth.
4. Pour this mixture into the pot and add Thai red curry paste, vegetable broth, coconut milk, and pink salt.
5. Mix well and allow to cook for about 20 minutes on low heat. Serve hot.

Nutrition:

Calories 269

Fat 24.1g

Cholesterol 0mg

Sodium 807mg

Carbs 8.8g

Fiber 1.7g

Sugars 4.6g

Protein 6.6g

40. Cream of Mushroom Soup

Preparation time: 15 minutes

Cooking time: 40 minutes

Servings: 2

Ingredients:

- 1½ cups unsweetened almond milk
- 2 cups cauliflower florets
- Onion powder
- salt
- black pepper
- 1 ½ cups diced white mushrooms
- ½ teaspoon extra-virgin olive oil

Directions:

1. Put the almond milk, cauliflower florets, onion powder, salt, and black pepper in a saucepan.
2. Cover the lid and bring to a boil. Lower the heat and allow to simmer for about 10 minutes. Transfer into a food processor and process until smooth.
3. Meanwhile, heat olive oil in a saucepan and add mushrooms. Cook for about 7 minutes and stir in the cauliflower puree.

4. Simmer, covered for about 10 minutes. Serve.

Nutrition:

Calories 76

Fat 4.1g

Cholesterol 0mg

Sodium 168mg

Carbs 8.6g

Fiber 3.8g

Sugars 3.3g

Protein 4.4g

41. Keto Taco Soup

Preparation time: 15 minutes

Cooking time: 28 minutes

Servings: 2

Ingredients:

- 1 tablespoon taco seasoning
- ¼ pound ground beef
- 2 cups beef bone broth
- 2 tablespoons Ranch dressing
- 2 tablespoons tomatoes, diced

Directions:

1. Cook the ground beef on medium-high heat in the large pot for about 10 minutes.
2. Add taco seasoning and bone broth and cook on low heat for about 8 minutes. Stir in the tomatoes and simmer for about 10 minutes.
3. Remove from heat and allow to cool. Add ranch dressing and mix well to serve.

Nutrition:

Calories 136

Fat 3.7g

Cholesterol 51mg

Sodium 738mg

Carbs 5.3g

Fiber 0.2g

Sugars 1.7g

Protein 18.2g

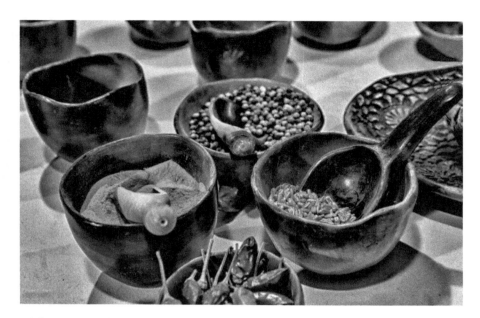

Chapter 8

Sauces, Dressings & Dips

42. Pepper Sauce

Preparation time: 15 minutes

Cooking time: 13 minutes

Servings: 1

Ingredients:

- ½ tsp White pepper, ground
- 2 tbsp Green peppercorns
- ½ tsp Salt

- 1 cup vegetable broth
- ½ medium Yellow onion diced fine
- ½ cup Heavy cream
- 1/tbsp butter
- ½ tsp Black pepper
- ½ tsp Xanthan gum

Directions:

1. In a saucepot, fry the onion in the melted butter using high heat for five minutes. Blend in the vegetable broth and mix it in well.
2. Stir in the white pepper, green peppercorns, and black pepper along with the heavy cream and let this mixture simmer for seven to eight minutes while you are constantly stirring.
3. Add in the salt and the xanthan gum and stir well and then remove the pot from the heat.

Nutrition:

Calories: 66

Carbs: 6g

Fat: 4g

Protein: 1g

43. Sweet Soy Sauce

Preparation time: 15 minutes

Cooking time: 25 minutes

Servings: 1

Ingredients:

- 1 cup Tamari sauce
- 1 ¼ cup xylitol

Directions:

1. Put the tamari sauce and the xylitol into a saucepot and set the pot over low heat. Stir this mixture often while you cook it at a simmer for twenty to twenty-five minutes.
2. When the xylitol is completely dissolved and the sauce is slightly thickened, then it is done.
3. You will be able to keep this sauce for up to three weeks in the refrigerator if you store it in a container that is completely sealed.

Nutrition:

Calories: 105

Carbs: 26g

Fat: 0g

Protein: 5g

44. White Cheese Sauce

Preparation time: 15 minutes

Cooking time: 20 minutes

Servings: 1

Ingredients:

- 1 cup Heavy cream
- 1 cup Butter
- 8 oz Cream cheese
- 2 cups Mozzarella cheese, shredded

Directions:

1. Cut the cream cheese into small chunks. Set a large saucepot over low heat and put the heavy cream, butter, and cream cheese into the pot.
2. Stir the ingredients constantly while they begin to melt over the heat and mix all.
3. When the ingredients have all mixed and become a creamy liquid, then stir in the shredded Mozzarella cheese and continue constantly stirring while the cheese melts.
4. This sauce will only need to be warmed again over low heat or in the microwave for one

minute to be able to use it, but you can only keep it in the refrigerator for three days.

Nutrition:

Calories: 38

Carbs: 2g

Fat: 3g

Protein: 2g

45. Marinara Sauce

Preparation time: 15 minutes

Cooking time: 20 minutes

Servings: 1

Ingredients:

- 2 tsp Oregano, fine chop
- 1 tsp Salt
- 2 tbsp Parsley, fine chop
- 3 cups Tomato puree
- 1 tbsp Garlic, minced
- 2 tbsp Onion flakes
- 2 tbsp Olive oil
- 2 tbsp Thyme, finely chop
- 1 tbsp Balsamic vinegar
- 1 tsp Black pepper

Directions:

1. In a medium-sized sauce, pot blends the oregano, thyme, garlic, onion flakes, and olive oil until all of the ingredients are smooth.
2. Set the heat to low and let this mixture simmer while you stir in the pepper, salt, and balsamic

vinegar and blend all of the ingredients well. Remove and stir in the parsley. Serve.

Nutrition:

Calories: 50

Carbs: 8g

Fat: 2g

Protein: 1g

46. Creamy Alfredo Sauce

Preparation time: 15 minutes

Cooking time: 5 minutes

Servings: 1

Ingredients:

- 1 Egg
- 1 tsp Salt
- 2 oz Parmesan cheese, fresh grated
- 3 oz Cream cheese, at room temperature
- 2 tbsp butter, at room temperature
- 1 cup Heavy cream
- ¼ tsp White pepper
- ¼ tsp Nutmeg, ground

Directions:

1. Put the butter plus the cream cheese in a medium-sized pot over very low heat and often stir while the cream cheese and the butter melt.
2. Adjust the heat up slightly and pour in one-fourth cup of the Parmesan cheese, frequently stirring while the cheese melts and blends in, and the mix is creamy and smooth.
3. Add a bit of the heavy cream and some Parmesan cheese, taking turns with these ingredients until blended.
4. Whisk or beat the egg in a small bowl and then pour it into the pot of hot sauce while you are constantly stirring to mix the egg in.

5. Cook the sauce for four to five more minutes while the sauce thickens and then stir in the seasonings and take the sauce off the heat.

Nutrition:

Calories: 60

Carbs: 4g

Fat: 5g

Protein: 1g

47. Lemon Herb Sauce

Preparation time: 15 minutes

Cooking time: 0 minutes

Servings: 1

Ingredients:

- 1 bunch cilantro, chopped
- 1 tsp red pepper flakes
- 2 tbsp lemon zest
- ¼ cup olive oil
- 2 tsp black pepper
- 2 tbsp lemon juice
- 1 tsp salt
- 1 bunch parsley, chopped
- 1 garlic, clove, smash
- 1 bunch mint, chopped
- 1 shallot, one, chop

Directions:

1. Blend the lemon zest, cilantro, garlic, black pepper, salt, parsley, mint, and shallots in a food processor or a blender until the ingredients are creamy and smooth.

2. Blend in the olive oil plus the lemon juice and stir until they are well mixed in. Then blend one more time after adding in the red pepper flakes. You can keep this sauce for no more than one week.

Nutrition:

Calories: 42

Carbs: 1g

Fat: 4g

Protein: 1g

48. Pesto Sauce

Preparation time: 15 minutes

Cooking time: 0 minutes

Servings: 1

Ingredients:

- 2 tbsp Garlic, minced
- 1 tsp Salt
- 2 tbsp butter, softened to room temperature
- 1 tsp Black pepper
- 2 cups basil, fresh leaves, chopped
- ½ cup MCT oil

Directions:

1. Cream the minced garlic, MCT oil, and the chopped basil until the ingredients are well mixed. Then blend in the softened butter and the parmesan cheese until they are mixed in well.
2. It is best to use this sauce immediately, but you can store it in the refrigerator for up to a week.
3. Before storing it, pour a thin layer of olive oil over the pesto to keep the top soft and keep the

air out. Before using it, just stir the olive oil into
the pesto mix.

Nutrition:

Calories: 80

Carbs: 1g

Fat: 8g

Protein: 3g

49. Cilantro Avocado Sauce

Preparation time: 15 minutes

Cooking time: 0 minutes

Servings: 1

Ingredients:

- ½ cup Water
- 2 tbsp Lime juice
- 2 tbsp MCT oil
- ½ tsp Salt
- 3 bunches Cilantro, fresh
- 2 tbsp Garlic, minced
- 2 tbsp Lemon juice

Directions:

1. Chop the cilantro into a fine chop. Then mix it with the lemon juice, garlic, salt, MCT oil, and the lime juice until the ingredients are creamy and smooth.
2. Use the water to add in a teaspoon at a time if you need to make the sauce a bit less thick.
3. Although you can store the sauce in the refrigerator for no more than three days, it will taste the best if you use it immediately.

Nutrition:

Calories: 50

Carbs: 3g

Fat: 4g

Protein: 2g

50. Strawberry Jam

Preparation time: 15 minutes

Cooking time: 20 minutes

Servings: 1

Ingredients:

- 1 cup Strawberries, diced
- ¼ cup Water
- ¾ tsp Knox gelatin powder
- 1 tbsp Lemon juice
- ¼ cup Sugar replacement

Directions:

- Pour the lemon juice into a bowl and pour the gelatin powder on top of it. Let this sit and get thick.
- Put the sugar replacement, water, and the strawberries into a small saucepot and then put it over medium heat. Then turn the heat to a very low as soon as the mix starts to simmer, and let it simmer for twenty minutes.
- While the mix is simmering, chop up the gelatin mix and place it in the warm strawberry mix and stir until it dissolves.

- Remove and let it cool before you place it in a container to store it in the refrigerator. You can keep this in the fridge for two weeks.

Nutrition:

Calories: 60

Carbs: 14g

Fat: 0g

Protein: 0g

Conclusion

Congratulations on making it through this part! It only means that you have greatly impacted your healthy lifestyle as a woman after her 50's by gaining all the knowledge about Keto Diet and how you can benefit from it.

Many women want to lose weight, but women over the age of 50 are particularly interested in losing weight, boosting their immune system, and having more energy.

If you fit into this group, this last part of this guide will address the particular hurdles you may face when doing the Keto diet. For one thing, women in this age range experience slowing metabolisms, making it harder to drop pounds than ever before.

We will cover the tweaks you can make to your Keto diet and lifestyle to accommodate these particular hurdles. We will talk about any concerns you may have and give you solutions to counteract them.

Women go through menopause sometime between the ages of 45 and 55, which can be a particularly difficult time. They notice they are putting on weight, and they experience all kinds of unpleasant symptoms such as difficulty sleeping and hot flashes.

But many of these symptoms are temporary. The one that bothers women the most is the one that lasts: weight gain. Women over 50 want to know how they can stave off weight gain and lose the extra pounds they started to put on after menopause.

Women in this age range can still go wrong when they try Keto and autophagy, so we have some pieces of advice to give you if you count yourself among this group.

The first piece of advice is to make sure you eat enough protein every day. You might be worried about eating too much protein because you are watching calories, which is a reasonable thing to do. But when you are on Keto, you need protein as a source of energy.

It is always about balance. On the one hand, you need to make up for the energy you won't be getting from carbs. On the other hand, you have to be careful not to eat too many calories.

As usual, follow along with what your body is telling you. If your body tells you that you still need more energy, wait a bit. You can eat more if some time passes and you still feel hungry. That probably means you need energy food. But you have to give yourself this waiting period because otherwise, your mind might be trying to trick you into just eating something you are craving when you are not genuinely hungry.

There is a mental component to this change in diet, too. The problem at the center of women not being able to change their diet is not being used to the real feeling of being full. By the "real" feeling of being full, we refer to how people feel when they have eaten enough—not too much.

These days, people eat so many carbs that their idea of fullness is the uncomfortable feeling when they eat too many carbs. But you can't lose weight if you see fullness this way. You will consistently overstuff yourself, believing you are making yourself full when you are gorging yourself.

To remind yourself what fullness feels like, get used to eating without overstuffing yourself. Get used to not feel uncomfortable after eating. It can feel strangely comforting to be overstuffed with carbs, but that is not a feeling we can let ourselves get used to. If we do, we will never be happy with the simple feeling of fullness.

As we keep emphasizing, we can't villainize fat anymore. The real problem is eating too many calories, most of which tend to come from carbs, not fats. However, in particular, women over 50 need to be careful not to eat too many fats when they follow Keto.

Keto isn't a valid excuse for simply eating a ton of fat. You still need to show some constraint as you do in every diet. Understanding how to balance your fat consumption will take learning how fat fits into Keto. With Keto, you want to be what we call fat-adapted.

You already know what this means; it is just another way of saying what happens in Ketosis. Being fat-adapted means you are burning fat for energy with Ketones instead of burning glucose with carbs.

We tell you this term because you should eat many healthy fats until you go through significant Ketosis — until you are fat-adapted. Once that happens, you should start being more careful with how much fat you are consuming.

One of the sources women over 50 will get fat from is drinks. Even the drinks you make at home, like coffee with milk, can be a lot higher in fat than you think. It should go without saying that the specialty coffee you get topped with whipped cream is high in fat.

Women over 50 know they have their hurdles to overcome when they chase weight loss goals and improve overall health with Keto. But they can do all they can do by following along with the advice in this guide. So, all in all, you have nothing to worry about! We've got your back. Happy-healthy eating!

CPSIA information can be obtained
at www.ICGtesting.com
Printed in the USA
BVHW090328040521
606332BV00006B/1208